The

Runaway Learning Machine:

Growing Up Dyslexic

by

James J. Bauer

Copyright 1992
Educational Media Corporation®

Library of Congress Catalog Card No. 92-071009

ISBN 0-932796-43-5

Printing (Last Digit)

10   9   8   7   6   5   4   3   2

Publisher—
Educational Media Corporation®
P.O. Box 2131
Minneapolis, MN 55421-0311
(612) 781-0088

Production editor—
Don L. Sorenson

Graphic design—
Earl Sorenson

Dedication

To
Molly F. Bauer
C. Wilson Anderson
Sigurd M. Hoppe, Ph.D.

Table of Contents

Chapter

1

Preschool

My first memories as a very young child are as I expect much like those of other children. Glimpses of emotionally scattered events from our first house and those social significant giants known as parents, aunts, uncles, and older siblings. But my first clear recall of my first years came at age 3 or 4 when my family moved to an old farmhouse in Ohio. This is where I first recall being me.

The house seemed like a giant cathedral to me—a small boy. The ceilings reached to the heavens. The kitchen seemed ten miles from the upstairs bedrooms. The basement was a cold, dark dungeon where certainly the bogeyman lived and disappeared only when adults ventured down the creaky stairs. There was one room off the kitchen, cold and dark, which no one really seemed to know its origin or significance to the rest of the house.

There was an old, weather-beaten barn which at one time was red, with a hayloft that would enchant a thousand children. The lower part of the barn held cattle and machinery. Next to the barn was a pig barn which each season held two pigs which I named Sam and Cleo. Each fall, the landlord would board Sam and Cleo on a truck only to return the following spring—a bit smaller. In my small boy's mind,, these were the same pigs, Sam and Cleo.

There was a large machinery shed built of cement blocks, younger than the other buildings, which held a wealth of old farm equipment including a horse-drawn buggy that could mesmerize a child. The attic of the machine shed was filled with old fruit baskets from the farm's better days, and when broken up, they made wondrous toy glider airplanes.

Closer to the house was a small building called the milkhouse which was no longer used as such, but was filled with my father's tools. Next to the milkhouse was an old windmill which had long ago lost its function, but it stood like a giant reaching as high as a mountain.

The entire farmyard was surrounded by a split rail fence. One part appeared to me, a small boy, to be a horse. The split rail fence horse's name was Ross. The front yard was shaded by two huge maple trees that each spring were tapped to collect their marvelous sap.

There was no kindergarten to go to, but that did not seem to bother anyone, least of all myself. This farming area had no such luxury, so I continued to learn and to explore the world on my own. With the help of peers who lived on the neighboring farm, I was very happy. All the fairs and theme parks in the universe could not hold a candle to what a small boy's imagination could make out of this old, run down, dilapidated farm. I felt as if I was where I should be, in tune with my family, peers, animals, and the world. The world was my oyster; everything was in balance.

But in the next few months, my world was to shatter. The experiences of the next few months would set the tone of my life for the next twelve years. I remember my mother receiving the phone call from the landlord; the farm was sold.

We had a short time to remove ourselves. I remember my mother crying. We had to leave the house. The house—the world I knew—was to be left behind. All of my days of building haylofts and catching snapping turtles were to be terminated for a life in the city.

It was about this time I remember my mother calling me to the living room for my first encounter with structured learning. She sat me down in a big, overstuffed armchair. She stated that soon I was to enter the first grade, and I would be expected to know my colors.

I squirmed in my chair as she slowly started around the room. The drapes are white. The walls are green. The carpet is brown. She repeated this a number of times, then asked me, "What color are the drapes?" I had no idea. We went around the room again. I was unable to succeed with any of her questions. With my squirming and crying, I was finally able to convince her I had to go use the bathroom; I received a reprieve from her. As I reflect on this experience in my life, I can only recall the living room as black and white. It was as if I was living in a black and white world; my central nervous system did not yet integrate color.

Despite this first horrible experience in structured learning, I still considered myself a fairly intelligent young lad. After all, I knew many songs; I knew about cowboys and dinosaurs. I knew how to climb maple trees; I knew how to pick apples. Skills such as reading and writing seemed like handy skills and nice tricks to show off with an aunt and uncle.

I thought I would have little trouble mastering such skills because my brother had mastered them quickly and was at the top of his class. I recall him returning home with his report card and, with the exception of penmanship, he received all As and Bs. I could not wait for the time I would be able to bring home a report card.

June turned into July and July into August. The time finally came for the big move. It was time to take all of our belongings and leave behind the old farm and move to a strange city house. I remember how much larger the rooms looked without their furniture, and how strange my brother's and my bedroom looked when the mattress was gone, leaving only the frame of the bed. I recall looking back at the old farm from the back seat of our car for the last time. I thought the house and the barn were crying as if they were sad to see us go.

Our new house was not too far away. It was in a small town, a village rather, called Aquila. It was named after an Indian chief, I was told. The house was pink. It was small, with a stone fireplace which was covered with a black piece of metal because it did not work. The front porch was winterized so it could be used all year round, with a lift-up trap door that led to the basement. The roads in the village were gravel, with a county highway at one end and a small lake at the other.

The village seemed to have many children, but for the first time, I was a new kid on the block. We lived in the village less than one year, a short time in the way an adult perceives time, but to a small child, it seemed like an eternity. This time would make great impact on my life.

I recall going on a picnic with my family, my aunt, my uncle, and my four cousins. It must have been Labor Day. I recall being excited because I could not wait to start school. I could not wait to raise my hand to answer the teacher's questions and to show how smart I was.

That night when I went to bed, I recall being so excited about school that I dozed off and started to dream about my coming adventure. I quickly sat up in bed raising my hand as if I was already in school. I was very excited about school at that moment, but little did I know that it was the last time I would feel positive about structured learning for the next twelve years.

Chapter

2

The First Grade

That morning we arose early. Mother was going to take us to school in Chardon, Ohio for the first time. The school looked mammoth, with my classroom up the gigantic stairs. I recall the smell of the old school. I can't quite describe it, but a smell my memory knows well to this day. It makes me want to vomit. My mother brought me to the classroom and introduced herself to the teacher, and then she told the teacher my name. She bid me adieu, leaving me in a panic, breaking my umbilical cord in this strange place.

The teacher hustled me to a chair and table called "your desk," and did the same with a mounting number of other children. This woman seemed gargantuan. When the classroom was finally in some sort of order, she brought herself to the front of the room and identified herself as our teacher, Mrs. Taylor. She talked about the day—lunch, recess, taking the bus, learning songs, numbers, spelling, and three reading groups.

I started to relax and found the lights in the ceiling interesting. I had never seen such lights, so I spent some time mesmerized by them. The teacher then demanded my attention, asking me what I was doing, to which I replied, "Looking at the lights", because that, indeed, was what I was doing. "We don't look at the lights while in school," was her response, which I found somewhat amusing. "We don't look at the lights." So she must have been looking at the lights too.

The next thing that happened I hoped did not happen in this manner, but in my reflection this is what took place. She went to the blackboard and started to write words "the" "and," "cat," "dog," "Jerry," until she had a list that seemed two stories high and 100 feet long. She went through the list a second time.

Then she talked about three reading groups—"the bunnies," the highest reading group, "the squirrels," the middle, and "the bluebirds," being the lowest. She further stated that she was going to divide us into three groups. After seeing which level we were on, she would further arrange the groups. Then she read our names and we were to remember our group. I was placed in the middle group.

It seems as if the next day we were expected to read. She went through the list of words again, then called us back in our specific groups. I thought I was going to do well. We opened our *Jerry and Alice Readers* and, one by one, each was expected to read a page.

It was finally my turn. I turned the page and was faced with something that looked like a neuro-anatomy textbook for a giant written in Greek. I fumbled with the book and had no idea how to attack the words. In silence I sat there. . . a silence that seemed at least an eternity. Finally the teacher told me the first word, then the second, the third, the fourth, and so on. Finally I recognized a word—"Jerry." But after that, I knew none of the words. Finally the page was done.

The teacher began to berate me. "You only knew one word on that entire page!" She was angry. I felt as if I was to blame, as if I had done something wrong. Her scolding seemed to last for hours. It cut right through me, taking all my self-worth with it. She finished by saying she was going to move me to the :"Bluebird" group, the lowest in the class.

Already the buzz was in the air that the Bluebird reading group was for the dummies, children who were not very smart. It seemed that the teacher did not like the children in the Bluebird reading group; so, she must not like me.

That night I was glad to be home. I played with my friends and later I ate dinner. After dinner, I was playing in the living room when my mother received a call from Mrs. Taylor. I remember the expression on her face as Mrs. Taylor laid out the gory details.

My mother hung up the phone, turned to me and started to yell, "Why aren't you reading? The teacher says all you do is stare at the ceiling!" She demanded that I try harder. I again felt cut to the core. I was bad. Something was wrong with me. I was an unworthy person because of my inability to please.

How could the other children learn to read and I couldn't? What was their secret? Maybe I can't read because the teacher doesn't like me. Maybe if I tried harder to get her to like me, I'd learn to read. It is strange what goes on in a child's mind when he feels he is not pleasing all those big people. Strange, but very real to a small child.

I recall a huge pencil that was black. This was the instrument we were to use to learn how to communicate the English language. I can recall being allowed to trace the letter "A." The letter had parts which were missing and we were to take our big, black pencils and fill in the lines. Then next to it, we were to reconstruct the "A" by ourselves. We went on to trace the remainder of the alphabet. I found myself fairly successful at this and it seemed fairly easy.

Then one day the teacher announced that we all knew the alphabet. We were expected to be able to construct the letters on our own. For most of the children, she was right, but for others, we were allowed to flounder, trying desperately to catch up with a runaway learning machine.

I remember sensing the anger rising in the teacher that some of us were not pleasing her, and we were not absorbing the information which she was spooning out to us. Strange things seemed to be happening socially in the classroom. There was a strange buzz in the air as to who was smart and who was dumb. The boy who was my friend on the first day of school was no longer my friend because he was much more successful at the runaway learning machine than I.

At recess and lunch, the social groups became more defined. Strange camaraderie when one feels rejected; he will find others that feel similar. The question was never asked, "Do you feel rejected? Outcasts? Or of less value?" But we had little trouble finding each other.

Then came learning numbers. I recall learning my own method of identifying numbers after what seemed like hours of the teacher drilling me. I was able to memorize, with the help of my ten fingers, the numbers one through ten. Then a small light came on. The numbers that started with the letter "two" always sounded like "two." You could say "twenty," then the number that followed, and so on, except for the teens. I then memorized eleven, twelve, then another little light came on in my head. When saying the numbers between thirteen and nineteen, you say the second number's name first. I was finally able to please the teacher. Maybe now she will like me.

Finally, it is time for the teacher to read to us—the part of the day I loved the best. Not because it came right before the time we returned home, but because I could visualize everything that she had to say.

Then, one day our teacher was not in school. There was a substitute. She acted nice and my thoughts were that she must like me. She read us a story, which I thought was great.

Then she passed out papers and asked us to write seven sentences. Seven sentences seemed seven hundred words long.

I managed to write one sentence, "I see Jerry." I pounded my mind for a second, but the second sentence would not come. Then, in my own creative way, I decided to write, "I see Alice." Then I wrote, "I see Spot." "I see baby." "I see mother." "I see father." "I see Tommy," and so on. I thought I was a genius. I was able to finish the project. I stood up and proudly walked to her desk and placed the paper before her. She thanked me and I returned to my desk and began to color.

Some time later, it was time for the parent/teacher conferences. My mother went. I waited at home for what seemed like hours. I hoped by some miracle that the news would be good, but of course it was not. When my mother returned home, I was confronted about my inability to catch the runaway learning machine. Then at the finale, she took out my paper with the seven sentences on it, the one I thought I had done so well. It had all kinds of red marks on it. It was not satisfactory. I again felt angry, frustrated, worthless, but above all I felt betrayed by the substitute teacher who cheerfully accepted and thanked me for the work.

Finally, spring arrived and everyone knew that summer vacation was near—a time when I would not have to deal with that concentration camp called school. Before summer vacation, the teacher had to fulfill a classroom requirement, and that was for the students to create a large mural. She showed us how to draw a tree. First you draw the trunk, then you start at the bottom and begin to draw the branches, bringing them all the way from the bottom up, becoming the branches.

We all practiced with our color crayons, and then when the teacher felt we were ready, she led us to the huge piece of paper, brushes, and water colors. My friend started with his brush the wrong way. The teacher's voice shattered the classroom, "Not that way! The way I showed you." My friend stopped, thought, and restarted the activity the way the teacher demanded. "That's better," was her reply. What was the teacher doing? We knew more about trees than she did. We climbed trees, we hung from trees, we built houses in trees, we fell out of trees. She was saying, "Don't draw your tree, draw my tree." So we did.

The last day of school seemed a week long. I couldn't wait to be free; however, I felt a strange feeling when the teacher said goodbye. I felt sad—sad because I felt as if I could not make her like me.

As far as the small minority group that could not catch the runaway learning machine, I wonder what happened to them. I wonder how many seeds were sown for alcoholism, suicide, marital problems, and basically frustrating lives. After all, frustrated and angry children become frustrated and angry adults, and frustrated and angry adults do frustrated and angry things.

Chapter

3

Return to Minnesota

The summer following the first grade was particularly stormy for our family. My parents had decided to move back to Minnesota where our family roots were. I recall saying goodbye to all my friends, promising them never to forget them. We were invited to one particular family's house—good friends of our family—named Romero. They were a warm, Italian family known to our family for their marvelous spaghetti. One of the children's name was Chris, and we were the same age and shared many childhood experiences.

We were in the living room when Chris brought a book about cowboys. He said, "I can read this. You read it to me now. You read it out loud." I looked at the book. I had no idea what the words had to say. His father was in the same room and overheard the conversation, He started to question me. "Can't you read this book? You and Chris are the same age and you're in the same grade. Chris can read this entire book. Can't you read it?"

I felt frozen, angry at the two of them for embarrassing me. I did the only thing I thought I could at the moment—I turned and silently walked away. Much like the experiences in school, I felt different than Chris now—different because he had learned to read and I could not. I wanted things to be the same as before, before I entered school, but now I felt that I was different than Chris. I felt as if we could no longer be friends. I felt glad that we were moving back to Minnesota.

The moving van arrived early the next day. Again I saw the house stripped naked of all its belongings. We spent the last night at our aunt and uncle's house because nearly everything we owned was in the back of a truck heading towards Minnesota, or in the back of a small trailer attached behind the car.

I remember lying in bed in the dark and saying goodbye to all my cousins. I had a sad, hollow feeling in my gut because I would not see them again for a long, unknown period of time.

The next morning came too early. I was awakened, and as my cousins were still asleep, I was hustled to the living room when it was still dark. I recall shaking my uncle's mighty hand. His muscular grasp almost hurt me. As we stepped off the front porch, my uncle said, "Look, there's Sputnik!" We all stood in silence, watching until it was out of sight. Bidding a final goodbye, we got into the car and drove away in silence.

The three-day drive to Minnesota seemed to last three weeks. I was unsure of my future, but at this point, I had little anxiety. After all, I was with my family; it was summer and that meant freedom from school.

Finally we arrived in Minnesota. We had made it. The old Ford, a rented trailer, a mother, a father, two sons, two parakeets, and a turtle. We had planned to stay with my aunt and uncle and their three children in a two-bedroom apartment for a few days until my father got settled in his new job. Those few days lasted all summer.

The job my father had secured prior to our move had dried up. The promising company had given the job to another man. Nine people living in a two-bedroom apartment made for a long, hot summer. Finally, after days of pounding the pavement and knocking on doors, my father secured a job and we were able to rent the lower part of a house which we found comfortable. It was situated on Como Avenue near the University of Minnesota. We moved into the house, it seemed, just in time for me to start school—the second grade. Possibly school would be different for me in Minnesota.

Chapter

4

The Second Grade

The name of my new school was to be Tuttle, just a few blocks from our house. I recall little about the teacher, my classmates, or the building because I would only be attending this school for about a week before changing again. I remember the feeling in my stomach—the hollow, aching feeling—as I faced all new people—not one I knew.

The teacher seemed friendly, as if she wanted to be friends with us all. She slowly called our names, and I anxiously waited to answer "Here." The classroom seemed immense, with ceilings which touched the sky. Big people forget how huge and overpowering a new situation is to a small person.

The teacher spoke of a cloakroom. The cloakroom? What is a cloak? I wear a coat. Oh, well, whatever you want to call it, I'll put my coat in it. Then she reviewed numbers. I was starting to feel comfortable. I already knew my numbers. Then she started to review the alphabet. I started to feel even more comfortable, because after all, I already knew the alphabet, but that was about all. I knew the names of the letters of the alphabet, but I did not know which sounds they made.

Then one afternoon I returned home and my mother informed my brother and I that we were going to be able to attend a Catholic grade school located near the University of Minnesota called St. Michaels. Everyone seemed excited about this. I had no idea how I felt about it. I guess I was supposed to be excited.

Again I entered the huge halls of another strange building after a long city bus ride. I was ushered to my classroom and introduced to my second grade teacher, Sister Appleby. She seemed like a giant, dressed in black with a little white collar around her neck and a little white something around her forehead, making up her habit. The only pink skin showing was part of her face and her hands.

She introduced me to the class, "This is James; he came all the way from Ohio." James? No one ever called me that before, with the exception of my mother when she was angry with me.

There wasn't a desk for me at that particular time, so I stood by the teacher's desk with the entire class staring at me in silence as if I was from outer space. Then an older boy brought in a well used, rickety old desk which had been painted black about one million years prior to my earthly arrival. I was promptly seated and I tried desperately to blend into the rest of the class.

One of the first class sessions was to be religion. In this class I did well because the information was, for the most part, presented orally and received auditorily. Feedback was given orally to the teacher, reflecting the fact that the information was retained. This lead ultimately to a grade on the report card. This was received well by the nuns, because it seemed that the nuns were particularly biased in the area of religion. If some young lad did well in religion, it may be a sign that God wanted him to become a Catholic priest, thus leading to ultimate brownie points in heaven for the nuns.

During religion the teacher would read the *Catechism* to us. We were to read silently to ourselves, following along in our own *Catechism*. I remember following the words, having no idea what they said, but I listened intently to the teacher, taking in every word. At the same time I watched the other children out of the corner of my eye. I watched how they held their books and I matched them when they turned their pages.

The second grade was the year the Catholic children were expected to make their first communion, so there was a heavy emphasis on religion. The second emphasis was on conduct. For some reason, conduct connected to religion.

I quickly learned that this nun had a habit of physically assaulting children if their behavior did not match her expectations. I recall the good nun banging two young lads' heads together, making a sound like that of two coconuts, so I was promptly stimulated to obtain an excellent grade in conduct.

It was strange how the judgment and actions of the nuns in the 1950s were not questioned. Their judgment and actions were infallible. The same actions even attempted today by any teacher would most likely result in dismissal and possibly even a jail sentence for the teacher.

Again we had the three reading groups, but this time we advanced to a new system—the first group, the second group, and the third group. The third group was the lowest. I was made a member of this group from the recommendation of my first grade teacher. In the third reading group were myself and the other students who could not catch the runaway learning machine.

This group, without saying, was not the teacher's favorite. Not only did it consist of the slow readers, but it also contained the majority of the students who acted out and pushed the school rules for recognition. In this new situation; I felt intimidated and shameful concerning my lack of ability.

I asked Jesus to improve my situation. Jesus will always help us, was drilled into our heads by the nun. Perhaps I was not good enough for Jesus to help. Perhaps I should be a better boy and He will answer my prayers. I recall one day the teacher was very upset with the third group. She lined us all up in front of the rest of the class, informing them that she was going to take us down to the first grade room and leave us there because we all were babies and should read better. I felt frozen and humiliated in front of the remainder of my classmates. I felt the young eyes looking into the depths of my soul, as if I was naked.

One of the children became hysterical. He was crying and sobbing, "I'm sorry, Sister," he said, "I'll do better. I'll learn to read better. Don't send me down to that place." The teacher finally allowed him to return to his desk. She further stated that it was obvious that he was sorry and that God had forgiven him. How did this woman know that God had forgiven him? This nun appeared to have some sort of hotline to the Deity. There was talk among the other nuns that this nun was a walking saint. This being so, we must have had it coming and everything that she said must be true.

I recall the nun having several little stamp angels that she would stamp upon our papers according to how we performed. I remember the lad in front of me receiving all good angels, an angel with a happy smiling face. I recall receiving mostly a sad-looking angel with the words under it, "Try harder." Try harder. Words that would make up the majority of my psychological script for years to come.

Chapter
5

Move to the Suburbs

The following summer still meant another move. My family managed to save enough money to place a down payment on a house in the mushrooming suburbs of Minneapolis. This was exciting to me, but it meant still another move and another new school.

The way the Minneapolis suburbs were mushrooming, it was much like a glorified shantytown. A bulldozer dug miles of trenches, masons built foundations for the homes, appropriately spaced apart, then the bulldozer filled in the remaining hole. Electricians, carpenters, and plumbers went on to finish the rest of the house. Hundreds of quickly built homes with basically two styles, rambler and colonial.

The city, if you could call it that, was completely unprepared for the population explosion, as well as was the school system. The nearest park to our new home was approximately a mile and a half away. The park, so far away and serving so many, soon became very territorial. If one from our neighborhood should venture unto this part of the world, he soon would be met with a gang of young boys who would challenge the turf, resulting usually in a fist fight.

Being very shy and introverted at this time, I shunned the park and stuck to my own neighborhood. I spent most of my time with younger children or watching the television. My brother, who was just as shy and introverted, retreated into a wooded area just behind our house to practice his scouting skills, or into the basement to play with his chemistry set.

The realty of living in the newly built suburbs was much different than the picture I had seen in my mind. But, still I resorted to my imagination to carry me through—an imagination which had its roots planted years ago on a small, dilapidated farm in Ohio.

Finally, September approached and the unavoidable became a realty. Time for school. The school system was completely unprepared to deal with the flood of city refugees to the suburbs. The grade school classes were split into morning and afternoon. Children from my area were to attend in the afternoon. Again, I entered a new school.

This time just about everyone was new. I do not recall the teacher's name because, again, I would be in this school about three weeks before being transferred to another parochial school. The new teacher seemed nice, a pleasant lady. I recall her talking about teaching. She said, "Some days when I go home, I feel like a good teacher, but when the children misbehave, I don't feel much like a teacher."

The school itself had no outdoor recreation equipment, again a result of the population explosion, so we just stood around during recess. There were trees but we could not climb them because it was too dangerous. We couldn't get down on the playground because that would dirty our clothes. So for the most part, we stood around and talked. School recess seemed long.

I recall the first time in reading groups. This time, perhaps by some miracle, I would be able to read well. After all, I had been praying much concerning this. Again, I was made part of the third group, again due to my previous performance. My stomach began to ache. My muscles became tight. I looked around and saw other children in the same group. There is some comfort in numbers.

One by one the children in the group began to struggle with the materials the teacher requested. I recall the anxiety as my turn approached, then my turn to read. I struggled with the first word, feeling very anxious, very conspicuous, and very warm. Then finally, after an eternity, I was done. This teacher's reaction appeared different towards us. She did not get angry; she did not scold or attempt to embarrass us. She just stated, "That was fine," and we could return to our desks.

After about three weeks I returned home again to be informed that I was to attend another parochial school. This new school, again, felt overpowering. It also had that strange smell that schools have. My brother dropped me off at the third grade room, then disappeared to his own classroom. The classroom was empty. Little did I know that all the other children were downstairs attending mass. So I stood in the back of the room, waiting for someone to rescue me.

After what seemed like hours, the class returned, along with the nun. I approached the nun and told her I was her new student. She stared at me, and stated that she had no new student by my name. There was a silence; I wanted to vomit on her black habit. Then she said, "Oh, yes, you must belong to the new third grade classroom." Then she hustled me down the hallway to another room where I met my new teacher, Mrs. Carlson.

Mrs. Carlson told me it was all right to be new; she was new herself to the building. Then she hustled me to my desk. Mrs. Carlson was an elderly lady with a severe tremor, appearing to be a Parkinson type. This parochial school was in such need for teachers that they were able to somehow convince Mrs. Carlson to come out of retirement. She was also from the old school of thought which allowed teachers to use physical abuse at their whim. As I quickly deciphered, as she broke a ruler over the head of a student who was acting out. Again, I was placed in the third reading group, the least favorite of the teacher.

During this time there was some sort of study done by some psychologist which said, in effect, that the reason some children do not learn to read is that they do not *want* to learn to read. Well, this spread through this suburban parochial school like wildfire. I recall the third reading group being confronted by Mrs. Carlson's twisted interpretation of the study. She looked at each one of us, looking sternly into our eyes, and stated, "You boys don't want to learn to read. Well, you are gong to learn to read if you like it or not."

I recall the conversation I had with myself. "I want to learn to read, God knows I want to learn to read. I'm trying. That psychologist, he doesn't know me, but he's a psychologist, that's like a doctor, so he must be right. Maybe I don't want to learn to read. Why don't I want to learn to read? It would be fun. I must be a bad boy."

Mrs. Carlson's tremor strengthened, her voice became louder, and her color changed as she met with no success. Finally, we were allowed to return to our desks.

Before lunch, we were to attend mass. I recall having a dialogue with the Deity concerning my lack of success. One of my first vocational goals was to be a Catholic priest, but the nuns and teachers made it clear that you could not be a priest unless you did well in reading and writing. Did God not want me to be a priest? I feel a calling that said, "God wanted me to be a priest." "You would feel a calling," the nuns said, "If it was true." Perhaps God would perform a miracle.

The third grade was also the grade where we were expected to learn the written alphabet, versus the printed alphabet. I recall struggling with the written word as if it were a completely different language.

One day a nun from Iowa appeared. She was some sort of inspector to ensure that the quality of Catholic education was being met. We were warned of her coming and informed to be at our best. Finally, she arrived in our room. She addressed the class and wanted to hear us read. She first called the top reading group. After hearing them read, she responded with praise. Then she called the second reading group. After hearing them read, she responded with praise and "try harder."

Then, finally, she called the third reading group. The group, sheepishly with our heads down, moved towards the front of the room. We quickly shuffled, trying not to be the first person on the end, for this person was always asked to read first. Then she asked us to read, one by one. As it became closer to my turn, I felt my body temperature rise, then finally it was my turn. I prayed for a short page.

I struggled with the words. Four words into the sentence, I met up with a word I did not know. I prayed for someone to tell me the word. She said, "Sound it out." I struggled with what sounds I thought the letters made, and finally, a reprieve, she told me the word. This went on until I finished the page. The place where my body had contact with the chair was warm, and I felt as if I had a fever. I had no idea how the child next to me did, because after that emotional experience, I mentally left the room.

Finally, she had finished with the group. The inspecting teacher closed her eyes and pinched the top of her nose for a moment in silence. It was clear we did not please her. Then she took her hand away from her face, opened her eyes, and spoke. "You boys must try harder." "Yes, sister," was our response.

For three years we had been trying to catch the runaway learning machine and she says, "Try harder," putting the responsibility on us. Then she said something which sent a shiver through my body—summer school. "You boys should go to summer school." The feeling must be similar to that of a prisoner when his parole has been denied. The only peace I had in life was the time away from school. This inspecting teacher was sure that the best plan for me was to attend summer school. Finally, we were allowed to return to our desks.

Recess was a strange event at this parochial school also. There was no recreational equipment, but we were expected to run, play, exercise, and not get dirty. We were also expected to attend recess outside even when it was twenty degrees below zero. I surmised that the school had a philosophy that this built character, that recreational equipment was a luxury, and to suffer with twenty below temperatures would build strong character in Catholic children and make us all saints.

One day Mrs. Carlson called me to her desk. She was displeased with my writing. She grabbed my right hand and said, "I will show you how to write better." As she slowly wrote, she said the letters of the alphabet, "A, B, C," and so forth. In my mind, I was running. I was frightened. Would she hit me? If I told her, would she yell at me?

I could not take it any longer. I spoke in a quiet, timid voice. "Mrs. Carlson, I write with the other hand." She stopped, looked at me and said, "Oh, are you left-handed?" I was so shook up at that point I couldn't tell my left from my right. "I guess so." "You guess so, don't you know which hand you write with?" "This one," as I held up a trembling left hand. She grabbed my left hand and started over again. "A, B, C," and so forth. I did not retain any of her efforts. All I wanted to do was return to my desk and melt into the rest of the classroom, and wait for the final bell to return home.

Mrs. Carlson, however, had not yet launched her final attempt to improve my reading. It was my turn to read. Reading from my desk as I squirmed in anticipation, I plunged into the page of words, only to meet with an unpronounceable word after three words. Mrs. Carlson told me to come up to her desk. She then demanded that I face the class and read. Sound out the words," she demanded. I couldn't.

Then a small voice told me the word—a sympathetic peer. "Quiet," she demanded, "Don't tell him." I began to cry. Tears ran down my face. Still she persisted. "What is the next word?" The tears in my eyes made the page blurry. I wiped away the tears, but more came. Fifty pairs of eyes stared at me while I struggled with the written word.

Finally, after what seemed like an eternity, Mrs. Carlson said, "That's fine." But this time her voice was different. There was a crack in her voice. She must have felt a portion of the ridicule that I was feeling. Then she stated that I could return to my desk. I returned to my desk, putting my head down on my desk, placing my arms tightly around my head, trying to shut out the rest of the world. I tried not to let the other children see me cry.

I felt shamed, angry. Why did she do this to me? Was I bad? I wanted to run away, I wanted to go home. I wanted to be away from the unclimbable mountain of education. After this experience, Mrs. Carlson finally left me alone for the rest of the school year.

Chapter

6

The Fourth and Fifth Grades

For some untold reason, at that time the school system apparently did not hold students back for any type of performance. So I was allowed to enter the fourth grade. The fourth and fifth grades seemed to blend together in my memory. Glimpses of a belittling experience, my subconscious has chosen better to remain buried. Besides, by this time, I started to enter a world of my own—a world within my imagination where the world was a more pleasant place.

I do not recall the name of my fourth grade teacher. One of the advantages of attending a parochial school is you do not need to know the name of your teacher if she is a nun, because you merely address her as "Sister."

My fifth grade teacher's name was Mrs. Stone, who was somewhat of the old school of teaching. However, she had less of a need to humiliate and to physically abuse children.

By mid fifth grade, we were expected to have memorized the multiplication tables. I was again having great trouble catching the runaway learning machine. One of Mrs. Stone's approaches to deal with this was to provide one-to-one tutoring with another classmate in the hallway, leaving one open to ridicule when younger children would pass by.

Then one day, when I was being drilled, who should approach but Father Mitchum, a fairly tall, stoic priest who walked about in a Christ-like manner. What are you doing? he inquired. "Drilling multiplication tables," my tutor replied. Then he took the multiplication card from her and addressed me. What is six times seven?" he asked. I froze. My mind drew a blank. I had all I could do to respond, "I don't know, Father." His response was one of shame and he made a sound with his lips. "You must try harder," he pompously stated and turned and walked away.

I felt ridiculed and belittled. I had failed to please the ultimate person in the school hierarchy and that was the priest. I felt angry, angry at the priest, my tutor, and my teacher for placing me in such a precarious situation—an anger and resentment that I would carry into adulthood towards priests, nuns, and teachers. At that time I would not allow myself to be angry towards them, because they were God's representatives on earth, I was taught, and so I turned my anger on myself, retreating further into my own world.

One afternoon, I recall riding home on the bus. It was the highlight of my day because it meant freedom from school and freedom to do what I wanted to do. A classmate approached me. He said, "Bauer, why are you so dumb?" I was shocked at such a question. I had no response but to say, "I'm not dumb." "Sure, you are. Everyone knows it," he said. "Why are you so dumb?" I looked out the window trying not to hear his ridicule until it came time for me to get off the bus at my home.

My brother, who heard the entire conversation, did not defend me in any way. He ran to the house, telling my mother of the entire incident. My brother, attended the same school. For the most part he pretended that I did not exist while we were in school. He was dealing with his own problems at that time. My mother looked at me and said, "You better not be dumb," in a scolding manner. Again all I could say was, "I'm not dumb." Then I grabbed a bag of potato chips and laid down in front of the television to wait until suppertime.

This was the first time I recall not wanting to live. I had failed to live up to expectations of all the significant people in my life—teachers, clergy, parents, siblings and classmates. That night, while trying to fall asleep, my mind raced, trying to find a solution to the problem. I fanaticized that by some miraculous means, I would show the entire class and teachers and everyone involved that I was not stupid, that I was very smart. I also had fantasies of physically assaulting the classmate who called me stupid and beat him to a pulp. But of course, none of my fantasies came true. I thank God that classmate never spoke to me again.

Finally Mrs. Stone made her greatest attempt to improve my reading. For some reason she got it into her head that the reason why some people do not read well is that they have no idea what they sounded like when they read. She seemed to believe that, if you were a poor reader and if you heard yourself read, that somehow you would improve your reading skills. She informed us that the second grade classroom had a tape recorder and she was going to borrow it so we could hear exactly how we sound when we read.

The next morning she wheeled the contraption into the classroom, set it up, and one by one, she went down the rows, having each one of us read a page. I fumbled with the book, trying to count the number of children ahead of me, and then counting the number of pages to see which page I would have to read so I could practice a bit ahead of time. I squirmed and sweated as the time grew closer for me to read.

Then finally, it was my turn. I started out, "Mrs. Smith said...," then I stopped. I had no idea what the next word was. I became very warm, very shaky, and I sat there in silence while that crazy machine ran. Then Mrs. Stone told me the next word. I fumbled with three more words and finally came to a situation where I could not go any further. Mrs. Stone told the child behind me to continue to read. Then with great delight, she played back the recorder while I had to listen to my classmates laugh and giggle about my performance.

The next day, returning to class, Mrs. Stone told us that she gave the second grade class permission to listen to the tape. All I could do was pray that none of the members of the second grade class would recognize my voice and add further ridicule to my situation.

By the end of the fifth grade, I had devised a way of dealing with the multiplication tables. I had learned to count by fives. If presented with a problem, for example, six times six, I would count to six by five. Five, ten, fifteen, twenty, twenty-five, thirty. Then I would continue counting by ones, thirty, thirty-one, thirty-two, thirty-three, thirty-four, thirty-five, thirty-six, coming up with the answer—thirty-six.

I had to be very sly and crafty, because Mrs. Stone would not allow us to count on our fingers. She thought by the time we got to the end of the fifth grade, we no longer had a need to count on our fingers. So when dealing with math problems, I spent a lot of time with my fingers under my desk.

One weekday night, my father called me to the kitchen table. He said, "You are failing in school. Don't you care?" My response was "Yes, I care." He said, "Will you try harder?" And I said, "Yes." But the reality of the situation was I didn't care. I had given up. Five years of school and I had failed to catch the runaway learning machine. This was the first time I had ever lied to my father.

Chapter

7

The Sixth Grade

Summer vacation, which always seemed to last an eternity, finally came to an end. Again I recall an aching in my gut. As the time grew closer, I knew I had no choice but to put up with what an adult could walk away from or quit. Going to school, I was again met by the strange aroma which school's have on their first day.

I entered the classroom to find my desk and to be introduced to the new teacher, Mrs. Austin. A middle aged woman, she was somewhat stout with a faint southern accent. She was new to the school, just arrived in the area and was very glad to be teaching again. She introduced us to a strange faced young man—her son, Mark. She went on to inform us that we should address her as Mam, or Mrs. Austin and she would expect much from us this year.

We were arranged in alphabetical order. My last name beginning with B, I was placed next to her son. Somewhere during the first week of school, I recall Mark being called to the teacher's desk. They were whispering and casting strange glances my way. On her desk I could see a pile of Iowa basic aptitude tests—tests which measure your ability and aptitude. The outcome of this test was based on your ability to read and make small black marks in the appropriate boxes. We were not given the results of these tests because it was felt that some of us would become over confident and others would become discouraged, so until this day the results of these tests are only known to the parochial school, God, and Iowa.

While the teacher and Mark were casting strange glances my way, I interpreted them as talking about me. After a lengthy conversation, Mark returned to his desk. Indications over the next few days proved that my interpretation of the conversation was accurate. Mark began to assist me in my work and for the first time someone was going out of their way to talk to me, the dumb kid in class.

The sixth grade, for some reason, was also the grade that one quit reading out loud and reading was done out of the text silently by yourself, by the teacher, or by a volunteer student. There was less opportunity for me to be held out in public ridicule, so slowly reading and myself started to blend into the rest of the class. In the past everyone in the class knew who the high achievers were and who were the dummies. It was still very possible for one to be held out in public ridicule by anyone who decided to do so.

It was the school's policy that the priest handed out the report cards, an occasion which I dreaded because this person had the clout in the religious and the educational community to ridicule you in public and in front of your classmates as he wished. This term we were to have the pastor, Father Wilkins, a middle aged balding priest. It was as if stress and high blood pressure soon would get the best of him. For the most part, he had no compassion for low aptitude children or children who could not read. I always thought he would do better in some other occupation.

The room grew quiet; the temperature seemed to drop as he walked in the room. He always had the teacher leave the room. The person that administered the grade, then, was not available for comment or confrontation by the student who had to put up with this priest's ridicule. Stoically he sat in the teacher's desk and drew the first report card from the top of the pile. A gentle smile came to his face as he interacted with the first student. He pointed to different places on the report card and stated "well done" as he folded it and handed it to the student. The student was then permitted to return to his desk. This went on until he drew my report card.

I slowly walked up to the desk hoping that I would not trip. He opened my report card and pointed with his huge finger and said, "How do you explain this?" I had all I could do to get out an "I don't know, Father." Then he found another grade and said "and this," again I responded, "I do not know." He folded the report card, shoved it at me and said, "You must try harder". Then I returned to my desk, sat down, and felt as if I was going to faint. At this time I opened up the report card and looked at the grades, because until now I was filled with so much anxiety I could not see the grades and all I saw previous to this was a huge blur.

At lunch, as other children cheerfully exchanged report cards, I slowly tucked mine in my desk and ate my lunch quietly by myself. The food slipped down to an acid filled burning stomach.

Sixth grade was the year I was going to discover something very interesting about myself. I discovered that I was much stronger than my peers. This was very evident during arm wrestling contests at recess and playing king of the hill on huge snow piles. In the evenings, again, I retreated to the television set, potato chips, and koolaide which added weight to me, but I associated weight with strength. I, however, did not try out for school athletics though baseball and basketball in our school were very strong.

I found myself quickly overtaken in any feats of coordination when on the playground and I felt as if I could not compete. The only thing that I could possibly master was brawn. I became quite a volunteer for any school activity which required such things as lifting boxes for the nuns when they could not lift them. In looking forward to my life, I could only see physical labor as my occupation. I felt that my lot in life had been set in the sixth grade.

Chapter

8

The Seventh and Eighth Grades

In the fall of the seventh grade, I was confronted with a nun who has a reputation for being the strictest in the school—Sister Dorothy. In retrospect, I would say that this woman was mentally ill and was dangerous. Nearly every day she would verbally and physically assault students for minor infractions of the classroom rules. I learned nothing that year but how to avoid becoming physically and verbally abused. Needless to say, these abuses never took place when there was another teacher, adult, or a priest in sight. I assume we were too intimidated to report such activity to our parents. In the mid 1960s, the nuns appeared to have license to teach and to discipline in any manner they saw fit.

The only redeeming quality of this nun was that twice a week she would read to us for 20 to 30 minutes. My vivid imagination took in every word as she spoke. Until this day I can still recall how my imagination visualized the books that she would read. Sister Dorothy appeared to have a paranoid view of the world. She would, during the course of the year, tell us how fortunate we were to be in a parochial school and sheltered. After all, she said, the public school was no place to be. Students in public school, by her view, carried knives and razor blades for protection. I interpreted that this must be true since it came from a nun, and nuns do not lie.

On one occasion the class received a special assignment from the priest. The assignment was to prepare a paper. On the day we were to present the papers, Sister Dorothy stoically walked around the room looking at the papers. A look was covering her face that I have only seen to this day on mad people. She stated that we needed to perform perfect work for the priest. She picked up one of the student's papers and found a mistake, then she ripped up the paper. She went on to another student, found another mistake, and ripped it up. She came to my paper, picked it up, looked at it, found a misspelled word, tore it up, and threw it in the waste basket.

One student who had been sick for a length of time had a note from her mother explaining why she didn't do the assignment. Sister Dorothy picked up the note, tore it up, and said she couldn't hide behind her mother's apron strings any longer. By the time she was done, she had torn up about two thirds of the students' papers. Then she left the room, leaving the entire class with hung heads.

The priest then entered the room and demanded the papers. Each student called upon stated, "I do not have it, Father." Then, finally a brave student spoke in a shy voice, "Sister tore them up." There was a silence and the priest said, "Well, she must have had good reason."

At this time, in the seventh grade, a young boy was allowed to take gun safety training, specifically designed to teach young men or young women the responsible use of fire arms. I was very excited about this course. It was the first activity I really wanted to join.

The six week course was taught one night a week. It was exciting because all the information presented was in lecture form. There were small amounts of reading material, but the majority of the information was covered within the lectures.

Everything was going well for me until the last evening. That evening we had to demonstrate that we retained the information that was told to us. The written test was true or false and we were supposed to place the appropriate pencil marks in the appropriate places. I had all I could do to fill in the top portion: name, address, and so forth. Now for the true or false portion. I fumbled with the sentences, trying to make sense out of blurs. I picked out words which I could read trying to put together the writer's intent. Then with my best judgment, I chose true or false.

The next week's class was reserved for obtaining the results of the test and obtaining our patches. The instructor who made a poor attempt to impress us with his pipe and plaid lumberjack shirt, read our names followed by our scores. When he reached mine, he read my name and yelled, "63, what is wrong with you? Didn't you study?" I took the paper from his hand and said, "Yes, I studied," and walked away. When I left the room, I began to cry, hoping no one would see me. I was glad it was over. I didn't want to see that instructor or the students again. I was afraid of their teasing and ridicule expanding upon my already increasing shame regarding my inability to catch the runaway learning machine.

One library day as I looked through the books for something interesting to read—something not very thick and not very hard to read—I remember Sister Dorothy saying, "James, you should find something within your ability." She went to the bottom shelf where the first and second graders found their books. She took out a little childish-looking book about animals. I was hoping that no one saw her, particularly the younger children. I was embarrassed that she had to go to the first and second grade books to find something at my reading level. She picked out the book and said, "What do you think of this one?" I said, "Fine," tucked it under my arm, and checked it out, hoping that no one had see me.

Art class was a very unusual experience in parochial school. It was used to reward children rather than to expand upon their artistic talent. It was something that was stuck in towards the end of the school day if time allowed.

One art class had to do with symbolism in religion. I created three figures with crowns and a star which represented the three kings and Christ. When we handed in our art work, Sister Dorothy went through a number of them, pointing out two or three of the ones which she thought were very good. She did not know which drawings were whose. She held up mine and said how excellent it was, that it was the best that she had ever seen, and that it had all the symbolism a good piece of art needed. She held it up and showed the class. When she asked whose it was, I held up my hand and said, "It's mine, Sister." She looked very surprised and said, "Well, that is very good James." When I received it back, it had been marked with an A crossed out and a B placed beside it. I was convinced that this nun decided that I was completely incapable of doing any type of A work, even though it may be in a completely different related field than reading and writing. I was extremely angry at her because I thought it was the best piece of art that I had ever done. Yet, it seemed that she believed that I was incapable of doing any type of A work.

The end of the school year was slowly approaching and Sister Dorothy was looking much more frazzled than she did at the beginning of the year. All year long she had been saying that she wanted it so quiet in the class room that she could hear a pin drop. On one of the last days of school, she opened up her desk drawer and took out a package of pins. She pulled one out of the package and actually dropped it. Yes, you can hear one drop if you are quiet enough; we were foolish enough to sit there and listen for it.

The summer between the seventh and eighth grade was particularly rewarding to me because I had my first opportunity to work using my brawn. I was young, but considering my body size and strength, I was put to work. I was sad to see the summer end because at that time I could have seen myself working in this type of situation for the rest of my life, never having to put up with the runaway learning machine.

During the summer I had learned that Sister Dorothy transferred to another school, never to terrorize students in our school again. I was ecstatically happy, but being polite, I verbally stated that I was sad that she had to leave. I hope that this nun, at some point in her life, received psychiatric help for her particular problem and finally learned to deal with her infantile rage, I hope she is no longer working with people, particularly the impressive minds of young students.

Eighth grade was headed by a nun named Sister Nancy. One of her duties in addition to teaching was that of principal of the school. She was fairly even tempered. She seemed to have an interest in the blossoming adolescent.

This would be my last year in parochial school because, traditionally, parochial school ended at the eighth grade. Sister Dorothy's words still echoed in my head about the dangers of public school and how it was no place for those who were sheltered in a parochial school. Sister Nancy seemed to want to raise egos more than the previous nun.

She often sought me out to assist her in school physical tasks and acts that I excelled at. When reading was to be done, it was done silently, verbally by herself, or by a student volunteer. So this year I was not asked to read in front of the class.

During the winter of this year a classmate of mine burned to death in a fire. The entire family, with the exception of the younger brother, had evacuated the house. My classmate reentered the house looking for his younger brother. He obtained severe burns which led to his death one week later. We attended the wake and the funeral as a class. Stoically we all stood there with no sign of emotion. One of my classmates began to cry, but later he denied it, stating he was laughing rather than crying. In a strange way I felt that it should have been me rather than him. I had developed no sense of future. This was the last year in parochial school and the nuns had me convinced that I would be eaten alive in public school. I couldn't read, write, or spell. My social life consisted of eating potato chips in front of the television and my best friend was the family dog.

Family and relatives all knew I was a low achiever, so when we gathered for family events, while others were explaining achievements and future plans of college, I would retreat to the corner in silence with a plate full of food.

My fantasy life was becoming more vivid to me. I would fantasize something happening to me which would change my situation—God performing perhaps a miracle—but nothing ever changed. When the situation failed to change, I began to wish God would move his mighty hand and end my life.

One evening when I was attempting to mop the basement floor, my father grabbed the mop from my hand stating, "Don't you even know how to mop a floor? If you had to go out and find a job, you couldn't even mop a floor." I was crushed. "Didn't I even know how to mop a floor?" I drew the conclusion that there was nothing I could do, so I left my father mopping the floor and mumbling to himself. I retreated to the TV set and my potato chips.

Finally, the last day of school, the last day of the eighth grade, I had mixed emotions. Summer was upon us and I would again be free from the runaway learning machine. I, however, was experiencing much anxiety over the coming fall in the public school system.

The last day of school I was asked to attend the school board meeting because I was to receive an award. I could not understand what award I could possibly be receiving. I sat through the other students receiving their awards for academic achievement. Then an explanation about my award. Sister Nancy stood up and said, "There is a student who has devoted much of his time in school to helping us with tasks that we could not perform. This person has been very helpful to us all year. We call upon him now and extend our thanks. We give him this award for school service." I was extremely flattered. This was the first award I had ever received in eight years of school. I was finally recognized for some ability that I had! This award meant so much to me that I wore it on the collar of my dress coat for many years to come.

Chapter
9
Junior High School

The day before entering junior high public school for the first time, I was convinced my life was going to end. I was thoroughly convinced that the public school system was a frightening place where children carried knives and razor blades for protection. The nuns also had me convinced that the public school system requirements were higher than those of the parochial school system. I was sure they would not be easy on a student like myself. But the law required that I attend school and I had to do so. I recall the uneasy feeling in my stomach as I entered the crowded bus for the first time. There were many strange and unfamiliar faces. In my mind I asked myself, "Will I be ridiculed if I am asked to read and I am not able to: Will I be able to hide my shortcomings in this mass of young people?" The school bus made its last stop and it was on its way to the school. The bus stopped; everyone jumped up as if on cue and charged toward the front of the bus.

We were then hustled to the gymnasium where we were expected to stand in appropriate alphabetically-formed lines according to the first letter of our last names. Then we received our schedule, the schedule we were to follow for the rest of the year.

My first class—shop. Shop was my only elective class. If you did well scholastically, you were allowed to chose a foreign language. If you did poorly scholastically, you were expected to take shop. Again, here was discrimination between the scholastic achievers and the scholastic failures. Shop class was supposed to begin preparing us for a future in the vocational areas; foreign language was preparing for college. Again, I felt my life was being set at age 14.

The shop began to fill with students. The shop classes drew the students who scholastically did not do well . There was much acting out and playing with the equipment until the teacher entered the room and demanded our attention. He called our names and we were expected to answer present. Then he stated that we would not be working on the power equipment today. We needed to study about the machines first. I felt disappointed because I had already been working with my father for many years in the shop using the types of equipment that I saw before me.

He passed out huge shop manuals and told us to read the first two chapters. Along with these, he passed out question and answer sheets which we were to fill out after we read the first two chapters. Then he went to his office, closed the door, and sat down at his desk. I opened the book and I attempted to read. I did not know most of the words so I skipped them, looking at the pictures on each page, trying to find out what the author's intent was. I watched the other students to see which pages they were on to appear as if I was keeping up. This went on for approximately fifteen minutes until the students began to throw things at each other until the room was a mix of half the students trying to study and half the students involved in this miniature war.

The shop teacher entered the room and the war came to a sudden stop. All of the students began to appear as if they were studying again. Again he left the room, going back to his office, closing the door, and sitting down at his desk . A few minutes before the bell rang, he reentered the room and told us to finish our reading and worksheets at home. He bid us an adieu as the group poured out the door.

The next class was math. The instructor appeared somewhat disgruntled with our class. He stated that we were the low achievers and pompously stated so. He then went on to state that neither one of us had a choice about the matter and he was stuck with us for the remainder of the year. He said he would do his best to drill math into our heads.

Then, as the previous teacher did, he passed out books and told us to review the first chapter along with a series of question and answer sheets which he told us to fill out after we had read the chapter. He returned to his desk, sat down, and began to write. A few minutes later he stated that there was something else which he needed to tell us. He went up to the blackboard and made some scribbles on it. Even though the scribbles made no sense to me, I copied them down in my workbook, attempting to appear to be a good student. He then returned to his desk in the previous manner. I did my best to make sense out of what he was trying to say and the scribbles on the board. Finally, the bell rang and we were told to finish our assignments at home and we were off to our other class.

The final class of the morning was social studies. This teacher, as the previous teacher, passed out books, but unlike the other teachers, she spent the remainder of the time talking. She made the class appear interesting. She also told us about being good citizens. I was taking in and understanding everything she was saying. If the entire year and every course was presented in this way and each evaluation taken in this way, I probably would have learned much and academically, I would have done quite well.

Finally, this class was over and we were on our way to lunch. My stomach was tied in knots; how could I eat? But then again, the system was telling us that now was the time to eat and we had better do so because soon the time would be up.

When I reached the lunchroom, I encountered a smell that remotely resembled that of food. I worked my way through the line, doing as other students did, hoping not to appear foolish or drop my tray. At the end of the line, I was faced with another dilemma, where to sit. I finally found a spot and forced down the food into my acid filled stomach. Then we were expected to evacuate the room and find our next class.

In my case the next class was physical education. I was nervous because all of the other students had phys ed before and they were familiar with what was to take place. They had developed many skills which I had not had the opportunity to develop.

The gym teacher was a fairly short man, aging, trying to appear like a jock or macho to impress the students. He informed us that if we participated, we would at least receive a C. Then he asked who knew the exercise routine. When he obtained the volunteer to lead the routine, he returned to his office, not to be seen until the exercise program was over.

We then showered in the smelly locker room and headed to my next class, English—the class I dreaded the most. I was faced with a slightly tall woman who appeared a little tired. She stated that this was the lowest functioning class of her day.

She further stated that she would much rather be with her drama class, but seeing as how she had no choice in this matter, she would deal with us in the best way she could. She went on to state that if we gave her no problems and turned in our home work, we would be able to expect a passing grade. She told us that we would be spending time in the library and we would be expected to read four books during the entire year, followed by a written book report. Reading and writing—these two factors sent an uneasy feeling into my gut and stomach.

Finally, my last class of the day, science. The science teacher was an older man, balding, over weight and approaching retirement. He had a reputation for occasionally taking students into the hall way and beating their heads against the lockers. Evidence of which was a series of dented lockers outside his classroom door. He, much like his peers, passed out books and told us to read the first chapter, accompanied by a question and answer sheet. He then returned to his desk and shuffled papers.

Finally, the last bell and we were allowed to return home on the bus, after which I took my potato chips and went to my accustomed spot in front of the television.

As time went on, I learned that the nuns' preoccupations with students in public school carrying knives and razor blades were nothing more than a paranoid delusion.

However, I still felt a great need to hide my learning disability for fear of being ostracized by my peers and teachers. I quickly learned that teachers would call upon you to read if you appeared as if you were sleeping or not paying attention or if you seldom asked questions, so I paid attention and asked some questions. Thus, I became quite an astute listener, a skill which I still maintain until this day.

The end of the quarter, the time for quarterly exams, arrived. All teachers seemed to have the same philosophy— one quarter of your grade depended on how you did on the mid-quarter exam; one quarter depended on how you did on your final exam; one quarter on if you handed in your homework; and one quarter was very subjective, if you got in the teacher's hair or not. This could be the final factor determining if you got a passing grade or a flunking grade.

Finally, the dreaded day—the first report card. Haunting voices of the nuns came back to me: 'Public school would not be kind to those of us who did not do well and it would be very easy to fail.'

Most of my energy in school was spent trying to perform adequate work and attempting to blend into the student body and not be discovered.

On report day we received our report cards in our first class. As we moved to each additional class, we handed our report cards to the teacher who wrote in the assigned grades. Between classes and at lunch, other students exchanged report cards. They compared how they did in each class. If they did not do well academically, they usually compensated by doing well in shop and in gym class.

I put my report card in my file and shuffled myself quietly to each class, attempting not to be seen. I was in great fear of anyone asking me to see my report card. In my final class I looked back at what I had received for grades. In every one of my classes, with the exception of gym, I had received Ds. I was crushed; I wanted to run away from the runaway learning machine.

I was waiting for the bus quietly when a friend of mine approached and wanted to see my report card. I valued that friendship; I made many excuses why I couldn't show him my report card. He kept insisting and, after a long period of time, I decided it was no use. I showed him my report card. He stared at it silently and said, "Oh." He returned the report card to me and got on the bus. He never spoke to me again. I felt that I had lost a good friend to my learning disabilities.

In my inability to catch the runaway learning machine, what few friends I had in school, I was under constant fear of discovery and fear that they would all abandon me, much like my previous friend had done.

It was shortly after receiving this first report card that I was sitting in my social studies class when I was requested to see the school counselor. I walked to his office in silence. I entered his office and sat down. He stated that he was going to give me a test. He stated that in light of my past performance, I possibly had a problem with reading. This test would indicate if I did or not.

The test, as I recall, lasted about 20 minutes. After this visit I was told to see the nurse. She gave me an eye test. At that point she stated that I needed glasses and told me to return to my classroom.

About one week later I was again called to the guidance counselor's office. He stated, "You have a problem with reading." He further stated that I needed to do something about it. Strange, they were the school system, given the responsibility to teach me to read, write, and spell, but I was the one who had to do something bout it. I was the one who had the problem.

I was taken down the hall and introduced to a teacher named Mr. Ender. He is our school's reading teacher. This class would take the place of my social studies class. So, with my new glasses, I entered my new reading class. The class was made up of approximately 12 students in a room which looked like it was converted from a storage room. The class was made up of children with learning disabilities, retarded children, and children who had immigrated from other countries. All of us were placed in the same class because of our "similar" problem. I knew I wasn't an immigrant, so I started to believe that I was retarded.

Mr. Ender was a fairly young and chunky man. He seemed to have somewhat of a compassion for our inability to catch the runaway learning machine. I had a strange sense of belonging in this class. All the students were having similar problems. I had no need to feel embarrassed or intimidated by these people.

Mr. Ender's major method of teaching reading was a system he developed where a student would read a short story silently, find the appropriate question and answer sheet, and answer the questions. The questions were graded later by the teacher. This system assumed that you knew the sounds that the English language made and that you had no problem with your space visualization or figure ground discrimination abilities. With the further assumption that all a students needed to do to improve their reading level was to read more.

The school year continued and I became more skillful at blending into the wall and hiding my disability. Occasionally, situations would arise where I would be called upon to read. On one occasion I was expected to read from a book in front of the English class. The night before the class, I went through the entire page I was supposed to read and committed the page to memory, stumbling over each word and then asking my mother or brother the pronunciations of the words I did not know.

The next day I held the book in front of my face and pretended that I was reading, occasionally glancing at the class and at the book. If I was asked to read a page from a book at the teacher's whim, I would attack the words the best I could, hoping that a kind teacher would grant mercy and call upon another student. In such a situations I would feel as if I had a fever. I felt very ill as if I could vomit; I felt as if I was about to faint. During this time other students would point, giggle, or poke fun at me—adding more torment to what I was already feeling. On such days I would be very glad to go home. I would return to my spot in front of the TV set, still feeling the embarrassment and the pain, watching television, and eating the potato chips.

The teachers in my school seemed to spend the majority of their time trying to maintain some sort of order in the classroom. It seemed as if the classroom could be divided into three groups.

The first group could be identified as the achievers, the group that the teacher loved to spend the majority of the time with because, after all, they fulfilled the teachers' needs.

The second group would be the group that acted up, fought, make noise, teased, but ultimately obtained the majority of the teachers attention.

The third group could only be identified as the flounders, not the achievers and not the acting out students. They just sat quietly, did the best they could, and obtained almost none of the teachers time because none was left.

The school year finally came to a close. Again, I was allowed to advance with my peers to the next class. It was really unclear to me why I was allowed to advance into the next class. Quite possibly it was due to the fact that I took care of the teachers' needs by not creating problems or acting out. Nevertheless, summer vacation meant freedom from the runaway learning machine for three months.

Chapter
10
Tenth and
Eleventh Grades

The tenth and eleventh grades seemed to blend together. Possibly because of time or possibly because what our minds feel is too painful to remember we will forget. Again, It was strongly suggested that I take reading class and follow the industrial arts part of the program. After all, it was quite clear that I was not college material. However, I had little interest in industrial arts and my reading ability was not improving at all.

In retrospect, I compare this school system to a shoe store that sells two sizes of shoes. If one doesn't fit, we will make the other one fit. In the reading class, I saw many of the same familiar faces I had the previous year. The school system continued to embrace the same system of teaching students to read, even though it seemed to have no effect.

I never felt part of the high school scene. Scholastically, I could not make it and sportswise, I was lucky if I could chew gum and walk at the same time.

So, as soon as I reached sixteen, I obtained a job after school in a local grocery store. I enjoyed working because it was one of the few places where I could obtain recognition for what skill I had—skills that utilized my brawn. If it would have been possible for me to work full time in this grocery store and drop from school, I surely would have done it. But after I inquired, I was told the store had a company policy that no one could work full time without a high school diploma.

It was the summer between the tenth and eleventh grades that I made a decision that would change my life. My older brother persuaded me to become a volunteer at a Minnesota state hospital for the retarded. This was sponsored by a Catholic youth organization in Minneapolis.

The application came, and with the help of my brother, I filled it out. The application had some questions which I felt I could not honestly answer such as, "Are you a good student?" I put down average. As far as special skills, I had none, so I left that blank.

Then one day I was called for an interview. I was nervous, but with encouragement from my brother, I attended. I really had little to say in the interview, but at the end I was told I was accepted. This really shocked me. For the first time, I was told by someone that I was appropriate for something.

Later I learned that we were expected to live at the state hospital, making friends with the forgotten, retarded residents. Before we left, I met with the other teenage volunteers. They were all from wealthy families attending private schools—a strange place for a public school flunky from a middle class blue collared electrical worker's family.

The retarded residents with whom we were to work were unable to take care of their personal needs. They were placed there by their families or the court system. The residents were, for the most part, forgotten—placed in a people warehouse which we call a state hospital. Many of the state hospital residents had no speech or no significant skills.

I felt a strange camaraderie with these forgotten people. They didn't expect, demand, or want anything from us except to have someone talk to them and be their friend. They wanted someone to reach out to touch them and to show them that they are alive and lovable. Generally, the residents were fed and kept dry by the staff. Otherwise, the staff was usually found in their offices drinking coffee. The few residents who could talk were usually actively psychotic, hearing or seeing things which were not there.

The hospital consisted of approximately 12 housing units which were called cottages. There were approximately 15 to 25 residents in each cottage. There was approximately two staff people per unit. For the entire hospital there were approximately two registered nurses, two recreational people, one occupational therapist, one speech pathologist, one industrial arts teacher, and one physician who was on call during the day. A medical student spent the evening in the upper offices of the administration building, who was usually drunk, studying, or other.

The three-week experience, however, was very rewarding for me. I found other things to give besides my ability to lift heavy objects. These forgotten people in some way were very much like myself. They were living in a system that they had no control over. Society and friends had forgotten them, they did not understand the nature of their disabilities. They were given up for lost. People felt it was hopeless and they never expected them to change.

This experience left me believing that possibly I could become something in life and help these people. However, that would involve college and everyone knew that college was very much not in the picture for me. I decided that even though the cards were stacked against me, I wanted to attend college and pursue an occupation where I could be useful to such people.

Chapter

11

Senior in High School

The summer before I entered my senior year, I spent half the summer working with retarded residents at a state hospital—the hospital I had worked at the previous year. The other half of the summer I worked in the Appalachian section of Kentucky. We provided emergency clothing and food to the people in this area as well as providing a tutoring service to the young.

Needless to say, I spent my time volunteering to work in the emergency clothing and food areas. This experience strengthened my conviction that I wanted to attend college and to obtain a degree in something which I could take back to these areas and help the people.

The people I encountered during these summer experiences strongly encouraged me to pursue this path. Little were they aware of my inability to read, write, or spell. My talents were greatly appreciated, particularly by the permanent staff, because I could do such things as repair their automobiles, a skill which they lacked. I also assisted in arranging the food warehouse, something I learned to do while working in the grocery store.

The permanent staff working in Appalachia seemed to have their own built-in problems. It appeared that each one of them had some sort of painful story which led them to run away to Appalachia. That was why they were there rather than to help people who were less fortunate. Many of them had broken love affairs or were divorced. They came to Appalachia to work the chinks out of their armor and to lick their wounds. One individual was actually able to obtain a deferment from his local draft board because he was involved in such work.

I inquired about returning and working with this organization after I finished high school, but they asked me "Why, when you can go to college for four years, return with a degree in social work or something similar, and be of more value to us?" I replied, "I guess you're right." Little did they know that college was not really in the picture for me.

The group I went with to Appalachia was again from the same Catholic youth organization in Minneapolis. It was made up mostly of upper income, private school students who were high achievers. I felt out of place, but I really wanted to be like them. I said, "Yes, I'm going to go to college as soon as I finish high school."

Later that fall I invited this group to my home. When they arrived, they were shocked to see how small the houses were and how they all looked alike. They said how embarrassed they would be to live in such a situation. It was a strange double standard they had—these people who spent all summer working with families who lived in nothing more than one room shacks. With the exception of one of these people, I have never heard from or seen these people again.

When high school started again, my senior year, I again returned to work after school at the local grocery store, a place where I felt I fit in.

Senior year was filled with exciting activities for most students, such as the senior prom, but I felt there was no place for me. I had no one I really felt I could ask, so I worked on prom night, went home, and watched television.

The Viet Nam war was raging at that time, and the blue-collared red-neck attitude ran rampant in the area in which I lived. After some strong thought on my part, I decided to side with the anti-war people, but unfortunately no one else I knew embraced the same idea. But what one does not feel a part of, one does not feel ostracized from.

Once again, I did my best to blend into the walls of the high school, hiding my learning disabilities from friends, peers, and teachers. In reality I hated the school system for its ability to humiliate me at its whim. I hated its teachers and its administration. I hated the community I lived in for its red-neck attitude. The only place I could find any positive stroking was at work because of my ability to put up with work that others found inappropriate or grueling.

About one third of the way through my senior year, the system started the big push—what will you do after high school? The choices seemed limited: go to college, university or junior college; go to a technical center; or enlist in the military. If one started to work after high school was over, he would soon be drafted at age 19. I continued to plan to attend college, but that was as far as they went. At this time the school was giving aptitude and interest tests. Approximately two hours of testing which combined with one's past grades and performance would outline the rest of one's life. My interest tests showed high interest in college, but my ability tests and past performance indicated the complete opposite. According to my ability tests, I was supposed to be a heavy equipment operator. This did not set well with me. I continued to stick to my wishes to go to college. During the supposed decision-making time, we were supposed to make an appointment with our guidance counselor and inform that person of our future plans.

On the afternoon I was to meet with my counselor, I was very nervous. I entered the room and I was met by the counselor who had a huge grin on her face. She gave me a very warm, verbal welcome. She asked me how I was; she said how nice it was to see me. There was a pause and then she asked me what my name was. She said, "Oh yes, I have forgotten your name, but I have seen you many times." The grin continued and she asked me what my plans were after high school. I stated that I planned to attend the University of Minnesota or a junior college. She said, "Oh yes, that is very nice." I further stated that I wished to study in the area of social work and become a social worker. She then stated, "Oh yes, we need good social workers." She opened up a huge book, found my name, and followed down with her finger. She was looking at my grade point average. Then she closed the book, as well as her eyes, rubbed the bridge of her nose, and the grin melted from her face. I sat in silence for what seemed like hours. I knew what she was thinking.

She turned and said that I would not be accepted at the University of Minnesota. Possibly I could get into a junior college, but I would be very frustrated there. She said I would probably fail in the first quarter. I asked her what happened to my ability to choose the direction of my future. She answered by stating that the high school could not go along with such plans and could not possibly, in any shape, way, or form, endorse me.

There was a silence; she then told me to return to class and rework my plans. As I walked back to my class, I was filled with rage. A few minutes ago, this woman did not know my name, but yet she was in a position to tell me what my future goals in life should be. If she knew how badly I wanted to succeed in college, she would have had a different attitude, and not have treated me that way. I further thought that I should inform her that it was my plan and I felt that my future was nothing more than a crock of shit, yet what was I to do? I needed this woman's endorsement on anything I wanted to do. She had burst my bubble. I had thoughts of packing up and returning to Appalachia, but for sure I would have been drafted.

After school, I went to work as usual and put my body into automatic pilot while my mind raced, trying to solve this problem.

My only other alternative was technical school. But, what do they have there that would possibly interest me? The next day I obtained a brochure from the local technical school and plowed through it the best I could. In the area of health occupations there was a program called Occupational Therapy Assistant. I knew they had occupational therapists in the state hospital systems. Perhaps this was something that would interest me and I could use.

The next day I called and made an appointment to see the program. The director of the program was not in so I met with her assistant. I was told of the needs they saw for the future and the need for men in the field. I informed her of my past volunteer experience and my wanting to work with people. I was given a tour of the classrooms and an application. That night when I returned home from work, I filled out the application. My mother helped me by reading the application and spelling the words which I could not spell.

A few days later I met with my high school guidance counselor who was very pleased with my choice to apply to a technical school. She informed me that technical school was more at my ability level and grade point average. With that she scribbled something in my file, closed it, and placed it in her file cabinet. The huge grin again returned to her face as she told me that she was extremely busy and bid me adieu.

A few days later, I received a phone call to meet with the director of the Occupational Therapy Assistant Program. I kept my appointment and was met by a small, thin, completely gray woman. She introduced herself and asked me to take a seat. She had a file with my name on it.

She informed me that she had received my application. She thought I would fit into the program, but with the following concerns. My high school grades were not very good. All the classes were at college level and she wanted to know if I could keep up. I felt very flushed; I wanted to keep up, but could I? All I could do was state that I certainly would try to do my best. I was then informed that I would receive her answer if I was accepted or not by mail. A few minor things were mentioned and I was allowed to leave the interview.

Many thoughts entered my head; the high school would not back my wishes to attend college, but would support my enrollment in technical school. However, the director of the program had just informed me that this was college level work. It was up to her whether I was in the program or not. The high school kept asking what are you going to do with the rest of your life? The high school even had the local military recruiter spend an afternoon at the high school. He directly informed us that if we did not enlist after high school or receive a deferment while attending college or technical school, we would certainly be drafted at age 19 and sent to Viet Nam.

The friends I did have were accepted into colleges with few problems, most of them with scholarships. Many of my cousins were quickly accepted into technical school because they did well in the technical areas. Everyone kept asking me, "What are you going to do with your life?" Military recruiters were calling me, sounding very intimidating and encouraged me to sign up with them with no delay.

As far as my high school counselor was concerned, my decision was made and my file was closed. Deep in my mind I had this feeling of falling flat on my face, depending on whatever program I became involved with. I started to have thoughts of removing myself from the entire situation. I started to feel that my only alternative would be to end my life, much like a high school classmate did a few months ago. I tried not to think about the entire situation; I decided to take life one day at a time.

Friends or relatives would ask me about my future plans. I had the tremendous ability to pull myself together, looking quite confident in stating that things are still up in the air, but I'm sure they will work out in the near future. A week before graduation, I received a letter from the local technical school, I was very anxious about opening this letter. I felt my entire future was folded within this envelope. I finally tore the letter open and it stated I was accepted to the OTA program. My anxiety about being accepted was now gone, but it was now replaced by a fear of another type, "Can I make it?" For now I was safe. I had something that I was able to tell those friends and relatives, something to tell the local draft board, and possibly a career to look forward to in the future.

I went home and took refuge with my guitar. I found comfort within the music written and performed by such artists as Peter, Paul, and Mary and Bob Dylan. I particularly found comfort in the song, "The Times are a Changing" by Bob Dylan. Words written by these artists very much fit my situation and probably are responsible for saving my life from suicide or a life of madness.

Chapter

12

Technical School

As I entered technical school, my social life began to grow. I felt it was because I could play the guitar. It was during this time that I also had my first date. I finally gathered all my courage and asked a young student to accompany me to a concert my school was sponsoring. There was a young guitar player coming to the Twin Cities called John Denver. My date had never heard him, but she thought she would attend. We were in a small auditorium which was nearly filled. I was extremely pleased to hear his songs which denounced the war in Viet Nam, still an unpopular view at this time. It was exciting to hear someone share my point of view. After I drove my date home, I felt very good. I felt good because I was beginning to have some kind of social life. I was receiving some kind of attention from the opposite sex, even though I was heartbroken when this young woman refused to go out with me after this first date. Anyway, it was a start.

A great portion of my school training was on-the-job experiences and affiliations. We were to internship at three separate centers for different types of experiences.

My first one was to be at a psychiatric day treatment program. I did well on this affiliation because most of the work was done with verbal interaction. I received good grades and the staff was pleased with my insight and intuitiveness. The clients were amazed that I was only nineteen years old. If I could have stopped here and gone to work in such an area, I certainly would have done so. But the course required two more affiliations.

My second affiliation was in a large metropolitan hospital. There was a heavy emphasis on charting and reading medical orders which meant dealing with medical terminology—reading and writing. I felt a sense of panic come over me as I entered the clinic for the first time. The first assignment was to read several articles that evening and write a short report on it to be turned in the next day. My sense of panic strengthened as additional reading assignments were added. One of them was to go to the nursing station and read a particular patient's rehab file. It was the first day of the affiliation and it was already filled with nothing but reading and writing assignments. I started to feel myself become violently ill. I wanted to call the school and tell them I quit. However, I gathered myself together, picked up my folders and pad, and headed for the area where patient files were kept.

I located my first patient's chart. All the writing and typing seemed to blend together into a whirlpool. I found the rehab section and found the appropriate sections where my particular charting was to be located—a major accomplishment already for myself. I fumbled with my finger through the appropriate charting. As I made an attempt to read it, I picked out key words. At the end of each paragraph, I tried to decipher what the writer's intent was. After a few pages and a headache, I was able to interpret the writer's intent. I used many of the words the writer used in my own report. I found them written in the report. I copied them correctly spelled onto my own paper. It was a twenty-minute project for an average student, however, for me it took an hour and a half. If the amount of effort I put into preparing this assignment was taken into account, I certainly would have received an A . Considering my spelling and sentence structure, I received a C-. At the end of this day, I was completely exhausted.

When I met with other students, they were glad that the day was over also. They stated that they would casually read the assignments and write a brief report. I said I would do the same; little did they know what they considered casual reading and writing would take me all night, and early into the next morning.

The next day when I turned in my assignment, I was glad that it was all done. A few hours later I was called into the instructor's office. She asked me what they were teaching us in school these days? She gave the paper back to me and asked me to redo it. I had an overpowering urge to smack her face. That would get me out of this situation real quick. She stated you must have not taken your time. I replied, "Yes, I guess I didn't. I ran through it last night." I swallowed hard as my stomach became filled with acid and tied itself in knots. So, again that night, I redid the report which I spent many hours on the previous night, only to turn it in the next morning to receive a C. I was then told it was questionable if I would be able to finish this affiliation.

Shortly after this I was allowed to work with patients. The instructor was amazed but confused at how quickly I developed rapport with the clients—particularly with the problem patients. I was given problem patients—I am sure—to insure my failure to ultimately remove me from their hair. I was able to quickly establish rapport with them and gain marked changes in their rehab potentials. Again the staff was strangely surprised. How could I do so poorly in one area, but exceed in another? The week before this affiliation was over, I repaired three pieces of rehab equipment that the rest of the staff was completely perplexed as to how to repair. The solution was obvious in my mind, and I went to work. With some simple tools, in a few minutes I repaired the rehab equipment. Thus, with my abilities to repair equipment and establish rapport quickly with clients, I was able to pull up my overall grade and finish the affiliation. I was very relieved to be done with this affiliation. I hated what I had been through and my stomach was constantly upset. It seemed as if my stomach was going to become a chronic problem for me. I vowed to myself that I could never possibly work in such a situation.

My third affiliation was working with retarded adults and children at the state hospital where I had volunteered in previous years. There was another student who had been there for a short time before me. I was very familiar with the retarded clients so I had no problems adjusting. Previous students in this affiliation had dropped from the program due to the stress of working with these particular clients.

The paper work was less on this affiliation than any of the other affiliations. The first evening I was given a vocabulary list of words commonly used in this affiliation. I was to look them up and to write down their meanings, which I quickly did with the help of my medical dictionary. Other assignments were to build different pieces of adaptive equipment. I had very little problem building them. I felt very comfortable with this affiliation and with these patients.

I started to develop a fondness with the other affiliating student. She finally left, returning to her home state and to her boyfriend and family. I felt heartbroken; I reacted even though our relationship was not that intimate. Before she left, I told her of the feelings that I had towards her. She informed me that she had feelings towards me, but only as a friend.

It took me many years in my adult life to learn how to deal with any type of personal rejection. Very often when we feel unfulfilled and have low self-esteem, we look for someone to fill us up. But until we can hold up our own heads and fill ourselves, we are chasing a dried up waterfall with a glass with no bottom.

Finally it was time for my affiliation to end, which brought my entire program finally to an end. Luckily for me the final exam had a good portion of verbal presentation. The final score was based on my overall performance. It allowed me to pass. I was awarded the title of Certified Occupational Therapy Assistant by the national organization.

Chapter

13

First Job
Relationships
and the
Deep Blue Sea

I quickly learned that words "need" and "demand" were two different things when it came to the work situation. When I entered the program, I was told that there was a great *need* for Certified Occupational Therapy Assistants, but the *demand* was very limited. Very few outpatient centers or hospitals were hiring. What few jobs were open I quickly applied for, but was met with a handful of applications shaken at me by the employer stating, "Why should I hire you?"

I usually carried in my folder all the information I would need to fill out an application. I would copy directly from my information with the correct spellings of such information as, high school, technical school, and references. On one

occasion, however, I was filling out the appropriate application. The first side was a usual application. Then when I
turned it over, there were many lines with a brief sentence
which stated, "Tell us the story of your life, use extra pages
if needed." Needless to say, after I filled out that application,
I never heard from that center again.

Time went on, with no job offers. My favorite pastime
became filling out job applications and receiving rejection
notices, which attempted to lessen my pain by thanking me
for my time. Although they told me they couldn't use me in
their center at this time, they would keep my application on
file.

I finally obtained part-time employment at a local
handicap bus company. My job was to lift handicapped
students off and on the school buses. Finally, a year had
passed since I graduated from the technical school program. I only had a part-time seasonal job which paid next
to nothing. I had very few friends. I was constantly receiving
rejection notices from job applications. The draft board was
sending me letters which I decided to ignore and to resist the
draft. I began to drink heavily whenever I had the opportunity. The few friends I had were into drinking heavily also.
Upon many occasions I found relief in drinking myself in a
different frame of mind, or so I thought. Life seemed
extremely unfair, and what was worse, no one around me
seemed to really care. What time I had away from work, and
what monies I made from work, I either spent on alcohol or
food.

At one point I was between shifts. I came home and ate
two submarine sandwiches and drank a six pack of coca
cola. Needless to say, I was quite uncomfortable and I also
was gaining weight quickly. I was five foot eight and
weighed over two hundred and twenty pounds. However, I
continued with my music, teaching myself to play better. I
began to play professionally, picking up a few dollars here
and there at local night clubs and coffee houses.

Finally, after nearly giving up, I noticed a small ad in the Minneapolis paper for a C O T A in Menomonie, Wisconsin. I called and made an appointment to apply that day. I brought the usual information with the correct spellings and so forth with me, placed within the folder to look quite professional. I met with the administrator who talked with me for approximately an hour and a half. A few days later I was called for a second interview, something which had never happened to me before. I came at the requested time and was prepared to meet with a sympathetic "Sorry but we cannot use you now, we will keep your application on file." But to the contrary, I was offered the position.

I didn't know what to say. I asked the administrator to please repeat what he just said. He replied, "I am offering you the position, do you want it?" I said, "Yes." I was extremely ecstatic about the offer. I finally was able to fulfill my vocational goals.

The two weeks before I started went fast. I had to move to Wisconsin, find a place to live, settle some minor business affairs, and say good bye to a few friends. It isn't very hard really to say good bye to a place which you never felt you belonged. My move to Wisconsin didn't take much. My suitcase which I received as a high school graduation gift came in quite handy. My guitar and a few books were all I really needed. I obtained a sleeping room in the local town.

The clientele at the center was divided roughly into three different designated groups: retarded adults, mentally ill adults, and chemically dependent adults. This would present a nightmare to some, but for me I saw it as a challenge and a chance to fulfill my vocational goals. My supervisors were pleased with how quickly I developed rapport with the patients. Even some of the patients who were very withdrawn and non communicative began to talk to me.

When it came to doing my charting, I would take pad and pencil home, and work late into the night with the dictionary writing out my charting. The next day I would take my pad to the nursing station and copy my charting verbatim into the appropriate spot in the patient record. If only my supervisor knew how hard I was working at my job. I finally felt I was doing what I really wanted to do. I believed I was making a difference in the world of human suffering.

My own self-esteem was building and I had an expanded social life. Working in this center, I met a young woman with whom I became quite involved. We began to make plans to move in together. Then one evening she told me she did not want to see me anymore. She had no reason, but later that week I learned that she was dating someone else. I was devastated. I was filled with rage over the rejection I was experiencing. Much of the rejection I had experienced in my past seemed to slide forward, resting at my feet.

My friends could not understand why I was taking this so hard and they reflected upon old cliches, "You'll find someone else," "There are plenty of fish in the sea," and so forth. I finally made an appointment to meet with a psychologist to talk over my feelings. He helped me sort out my feelings and deal with much of the rage I was experiencing. We also dealt with the rage that I had from the past. But, little did he know that I was learning disabled. I managed to keep this covered during the sessions. The ironic part was that fifteen years later I learned that he too had a learning disability, even though he had earned a Ph.D. He apparently was as skillful at hiding his learning disability as I was.

During my second year of employment in Wisconsin, I moved out of the community to the far east side of St. Paul Minnesota, 60 miles away. I was able to commute to the job with another man who worked in my department. I felt my spirit would do better living outside of this community—the community where I once had a relationship.

During one holiday week-end while visiting my parents and brother, a friend of my brothers told me about a man who was a private tutor and who worked specifically with adults, teaching them to read, write, and spell. Without tipping my hand, I inquired more about this person. The man's name was Wilson Anderson. I was able to obtain the name and telephone number of Mr. Anderson from this friend, stating that I possibly had some clients that could use his services.

A few days later while at work, I was asked to stand up in front of a group of peers and read a piece of paper. I felt flushed as if I could faint. I stumbled over the words and mispronounced them. I read the entire paper the best I could. When I finished reading the paper, which seemed more like reading a book of Greek to the group, I commented on how poorly the printing was and how poor a copy the printing machine made.

That evening as I returned home, my anxiety and fear continued. I decided that I needed to do something about my reading before I would either die or go crazy. The next evening I called Wilson Anderson on the phone. He assured me that most of his students were adults. If I wanted to come over and meet with him, he would be glad to make an appointment. I also asked him if it was too late for someone my age to learn to read. He stated, "It is never too late."

I thought to my self that I really had nothing to lose and possibly something to gain, despite the fact that I thought I was doomed to be a poor reader, writer, and speller for the rest of my life. So I made and appointment.

The evening I met Wilson I was extremely anxious. I had spent most of my life hiding my learning disability. Now I was on my way to face the disability once and for all. Wilson first asked me what I thought the problem was. I told him that I was an extremely poor speller, not wanting to tip my hand all at the same time. He said, "Does it extend to reading and writing?" I said, "Yes."

I felt a great deal of shame and frustration come over me. Wilson stated, "You probably feel a great amount of shame and frustration about this entire situation." It was as if Wilson was reading my mind. "How long have you been aware of this?" he asked. "Since the first day of school," I replied. "I see," was his response. I am now going to ask you to do the hardest thing in the world for you. I am going to ask you to read for me, not to embarrass you, but I have to know what level of reading you are on.

I agreed and I started to read. I felt all the embarrassment and frustration from my past life come forward and sit upon my chest. What I was reading was not that long, but it seemed like I was reading an entire book. I could hardly believe that it was my voice trying to sound out and mispronounce the words. After what seemed like an eternity, Wilson said, "Stop." After some additional short evaluations, Wilson stated, "Did you graduate from high school?" "Yes." "Technical school?" "Yes."

"Quite frankly, I don't see how you ever graduated from high school. It must have been hell." "Yes, it was." I felt very relieved that someone was finally identifying with my feelings, recognizing how I felt. "Where were your parents during this time?" "I don't know." "Do you have brothers or sisters?" "Brother." "Did they help you?" "Some." "Have you ever heard of dyslexia?" "Yes, but I don't see letters backwards."

"That is only one symptom," he replied. Dyslexia is present in people with high IQs, but for some unknown reason they do not develop the ability to read, write, or spell very well. Has anyone ever told you that you have a very high IQ?" "No," was my reply. "Do you believe it?" "No," I replied. Then I began to laugh. You laugh because you know that it is true.

"But I don't believe it." "Maybe some day you will. By the way, you are reading at less than a third grade level." In parting I stated that I hoped I could improve my situation. Then I made another appointment to start tutoring.

My thoughts were mixed as I drove home. Would I learn to read better or will this be a waste of time? I spent many years in reading class and still I am not a good reader. Perhaps it will change my reading and writing ability and someday I may be able to go to college.

At the first tutoring session, Wilson pulled out a set of flash cards. I stated, "I know what the letters are." He said, "I know you know what the letters are, but do you know what sounds they make?" He said, "What's this?" I said, "A." "What sound does it make?" "A." "No, Ah." He flashed the next one, "What is this?" "E." "What sound does it make?" "E." "No, Eh," and so on through the vowels until I had finally memorized the sounds that the vowels make. Then we went to the sounds the additional letters make and the combination sounds that letters make together. This was all over a number of months. At first I felt greatly embarrassed. I didn't even know the sounds that the English letters made.

Wilson picked up on my mood and confronted it. You are feeling embarrassed, but you don't have to be. Only after weeks and months of tutoring, my reading, writing and spelling ability began to change. It took me months of hard work. Slowly this man was working a miracle. The local paper started to become somewhat of an interesting friend, rather than a piece of jumbled words. I no longer had to spend countless hours working *on* paperwork, even though I still put in much more time than my peers. I started to feel that possibly I had a place in a reading, writing, and spelling world.

On several occasions I felt that my brain became over loaded. It was almost as if my brain short circuited, unable to deal with any more words—writing or spelling. It was explained to me that in one way my mind was short circuiting because it was not used to handling all this information. But, as I went on I would find it more and more possible to handle more and more written information.

My reading level began to improve. Other things began to improve as well. Words—long words which once appeared to be long blurs—became meaningful to me. I could take apart words and make sense out of them. I began to notice when I misspelled a word. I would recognize this and look it up in a dictionary, finding the appropriate spelling. Articles in newspapers and magazines began to become interesting. Other things began to change as well. My self-esteem, which was almost nil, began to rise. I took on new tasks and finished old ones—tasks which I thought I could never possibly start or finish.

When one has as few friends as I did, it is difficult to have an appropriate yard stick by which to measure quality relationships. In the past I began to collect friends who I thought were my friends, but for the most part the friendship was lopsided. They took advantage of my openness and willingness to share. As I began to read and my self-esteem improved, my friendships began to change. My old friends no longer wanted to be around me, but I quickly made new friends and better relationships—mutual friendships. My excessive drinking began to slow and I began to eat less and I lost weight. The changes did not take place over night, but over months and years.

During long talks with Wilson, and some formal and informal therapy sessions, I changed my life. He helped me to deal with my feelings of rejection, frustration, anger, and rage.

Through tutoring I went from learning the sounds that each letter made to an eighth grade reading level. When I reached the eighth grade reading level, Wilson told me that he could not advance me any further. Any advances that I would make beyond this would be on my own, by reading daily. At the last tutoring session, Wilson said that he had never met a student like me. He had never met anyone quite as bright as I was. He was very sure that I would be successful. I told him that I thought he must tell that to all his students and he stated, "No."

I was nearly finished with my tutoring sessions when I met Molly. Over the months we developed a warm, close relationship. For the first time in my life I was told that I was loved. To a young man who spent the majority of his life believing that he was unlovable, this was the final ingredient which turned my life.

Echoes of the past sometimes still haunt me, but as I grow older and continue to change, the echoes become fainter and further apart. Dyslexia still manifests itself today in my life. I need to allow myself more time to read and to write—more time than my peers do. The Webster Dictionary Company stock must be doing very well because of the number of dictionaries I have gone through in recent years. My imagination is still very strong, which I rely upon daily to problem solve and to create new programs and ideas. A quick wit which once saved me from embarrassing situations now is mostly used to entertain, to become part of casual conversations, and to make friends and acquaintances.

Life has changed dramatically for me, but it is still not perfect by any means. I have little time now for television, potato chips, or alcohol. I have embraced life at its fullest and am now making up for lost time. I have no time to lose.

Chapter
14

Conclusion: Upon Reflection of the Runaway Learning Machine

As I reflect upon a lifetime of dealing with a learning disability, I encounter its discouragement and heartaches, as well as its advantages. Yes, the above statement is not a misprint or a dyslexic reversal but a true statement. When one cannot be forced, coerced, threatened, beaten, or seduced into conforming. The result is an individual who marches to a different drummer and measures the world with his or her own yardstick.

In my graduate work at St. Mary's College, Winona, Minnesota, I performed a research project in which I interviewed several learning disabled people in depth. Sprinkled among a lifetime of inability to deal with the runaway learning machine were several themes of positive aspects. Among them were the following:

1. The ability to problem solve or see solutions to problems where other structured problem solving techniques that were taught were ineffective.

2. Next to be reported was a picture-type memory, different than a photographic-type memory. An example of this in one case was the ability to see a situation which happened in the past very much like a movie. The individual was able to recall a situation which had happened many years ago, complete with the color of the clothes each individual was wearing.

3. Many had a superior verbal skill which, if presented with the situation, would be able to sell an anchor to a drowning sailor.

4. Finally, a skill reported by most, the ability of intuitivism bordering on psychic ability. This skill was not only beneficial to social interaction, but ranked high among the survival skills.

5. Among the mechanically inclined in this study was the ability to visually see a piece of moving machinery, such as an engine or transmission, in their minds. Once visualizing this picture, they then had the ability to completely disassemble, repair the broken part, and reassemble the engine or transmission in working order without benefit of diagram or drawn blueprint.

On the negative side of the study, I have coined a phrase which I call "The Dyslexic Impostor Complex." This arises from confusion within the mind of the individual who is dyslexic. An example of this situation would be: If I have the ability to completely disassemble a transmission, replace a broken part and reassemble it in working order without benefit of diagram, then why can't I read the menu in a restaurant? Another example may be: How come I can recall a situation in the past which took place 20 years ago, complete with conversation, colors of clothing people were wearing, where they were standing, but I still cannot read the same book my 7-year-old child can read? Thus the person starts to hide the handicap, mostly because of confusion, and becomes an impostor. This is the dyslexic impostor complex.

However, the most devastating issue that I discovered in my study was the issue of self-esteem. In the study, when I specifically asked about self-esteem as a child, an adolescent, and a young adult, nearly all in the study answered, "What self-esteem?" It is the issue of self-esteem that concerns me the most. It is my personal feeling that our self-esteem is simply how we perceive ourself in the reflection in the world's looking glass. In my study it seemed that the issue of self-esteem was the one single major issue that determined whether a person with dyslexia made a positive adjustment to the disability or a negative adjustment .

After my study was completed, I became curious about another question. If the issue of self-esteem in others was so embedded in the dyslexic individual's psychic, it must be causing great problems with other aspects of their lives. These individuals must be coming in contact with chemical dependency counselors, social workers, psychologists, and so forth. I then asked the question, if faced with a dyslexic person that had a particular problem, could the individual , such as a counselor or psychologist, identify that this individual has a learning disability and deal with it?

I developed the following fictitious case history of an individual who is a composite of many of the learning disabled persons that I met. The composite is as follows:

Bill is a 27-year-old unemployed construction worker who has come to your office for the first time. He is a tall, well developed man who appears in distress. The initial questionnaire which you customarily have your client's fill out prior to the first visit was left blank. When you questioned Bill, he stated that he wished to give the questionnaire further thought and fill it out at home. The insurance part of the questionnaire was filled out by your secretary from information Bill supplied to her.

When asked what brings Bill to your office, he stated that his life is a mess and has been for many years. However, it all came to a head two evenings ago when Bill hit his wife, breaking her nose. Bill's wife promised that if he obtained professional help, she would not tell anyone that he had broken her nose. She said she would blame the injury on a fall down the stairs. When exploring further, you learned that this is Bill's second marriage. The first marriage ended because of a similar incident. Bill reported to have been to a counselor during his first marriage and was dropped by the counselor because of poor motivation. The previous counselor instructed Bill to read a particular book which Bill never did. Bill added that he has been an active member of AA. Since becoming unemployed, he has returned to drinking but he felt he has this under control. Last month Bill received a ticket for open bottle.

When asked about work history, Bill stated that he started construction work shortly after high school. He was liked by the company and offered a higher position. He stated it was too much desk work and he would rather be outside working with his hands. Unfortunately, the company folded.

Bill's wife is employed at a nursing home as an LPN. Bill has one child from his previous marriage. When asked about his sex life, Bill stated that it is lousy since his wife switched to working nights. When asked about his financial situation, Bill stated that his wife handles the checkbook. However he knew that since his employment ended, their financial picture was grim. In ending, Bill stated that if he could just get back to work, everything would be fine again. Bill said he will return next week.

In this study, there are four incidents that indicate that Bill is having issues with the runaway learning machine. One is the initial questionnaire sheet which you customarily have your client's fill out was left blank. When you questioned, Bill he wished to give the questionnaire further thought and he said he would fill it out at home. Bill did not fill out the questionnaire. He skillfully worked around it.

The previous counselor instructed Bill to read a particular book which Bill never did. Bill successfully scooted around the issue and was dropped because of poor motivation. Bill did not have poor motivation; Bill could not read.

Bill was liked by the company and offered a higher position. He turned it down, stating it was too much desk work. He said he would rather work outside with his hands. Many people would rather work with their hands, however, in light of the previous situations, Bill has an issue around doing desk work.

The fourth issue is Bill stated that his wife handles the checkbook. Many woman may handle the checkbook, but once again, in light of the previous history, Bill has some issues around learning, handling numbers, reading, writing, and spelling.

I then compiled a list of 100 individuals. Among them were psychiatrists, psychologists, nurses, chemical dependency counselors, vocational counselors, social workers, masters of social work, special education tutors, occupational therapists, and a small group of non-professionals. I sent them a copy of this fictitious case history. I asked them to develop a problem list for Bill to work on during the time that he would be in therapy with them.

To my surprise none of the professional individuals identified a learning disability as a potential problem in Bill's case history. However, four out of five of the non-professional individuals identified that possibly Bill had an issue around reading, writing, or spelling.

I will allow you to draw your own conclusions upon my study. However, it is my contention that the untrained person's eye was better able to identify the issue of a learning disability than the trained professional.

If allowed to go unaddressed, the professionals would be treating only Bill's symptoms of a troubled life and would not really reach the hub of the problem, thus performing only a band-aid job—a disservice to the person who is in pain.

In a more traditional book one would expect to find the most current theories or cause of dyslexia. However, this is not a traditional book nor am I a traditional person. I will leave you with six theories that six individuals have about their particular inability to catch their own runaway learning machines.

1. Something must be drastically wrong in the central nervous system.

2. It is tied to developmental system. Example: Some children are ready to learn at age 6, others at age 9. We develop at different speeds. The school system seems to think we are all ready to read at the same time, the same age, and almost the same hour. If you do not retain the information fundamental for reading at that time, you will be learning disabled.

3. People learn differently. Example: Some people are visual learners, others are tactile learners.

4. Emotionally, the learning disabled person was not ready to learn. Example: Emotionally upset about a family situation.

5. The English language is so complex; it has so many exceptions to its own rules it is a wonder that anyone can ever master it.

6. There is no need for a theory; there is no such thing as a learning disability. Society puts too much emphasis on reading, writing, and spelling. You might as well have a policy that everyone should be able to play the violin by the time they graduate from high school. If they could not, they would be disabled.

Writing this book has been more than therapy for me. I trust that as you obtain some insight into the pain I felt as a youngster growing up with dyslexia, you will be more vigilant concerning how your words and actions affect others. Remember how fragile and impressionable young people are. When someone is not performing as expected, give some consideration to alternative solutions rather than just saying "try harder."

Learning disabilities are *real* disabilities. However, with patience, love, and special assistance, people with learning disabilities can learn. Feeling good about themselves— having positive self-esteem—is the beginning.

James J. Bauer
7630 Bacon Drive
Fridley, MN 55432

Credits

I wish to thank the following people for their role in changing my life:

Molly F. Bauer gave me unconditional love and support.

C. Wilson Anderson taught me to read, write, and spell.

Sigurd M. Hoppe, Ph.D. encouraged me to write this book.

Non Credits

I wish to extend non-credit to the following for their lack of understanding and apathy in dealing with my dyslexia:

- The public school system, its boards, administrators, counselors, and teachers.
- The parochial school system and parochial youth organizations.
- State and national organization focusing on learning disabilities whose first priority is to maintain their status quo.
- Universities, colleges, and technical centers who refuse to recognize learning disabilities or dyslexia.

James J. Bauer